MEN – ~~O~~ TAKE – PAUSE

THE TRUTH ABOUT MENOPAUSE
AND MAN'S ONLY HOPE FOR SURVIVING IT

SUSAN CLARIDGE

Men -Take- O - Pause

Global Publishing Group LLC

Copyright © 2019 by S.R.Claridge

All rights reserved. In accordance with the U.S.Copyright Act of 1976, the scanning, uploading, and electronic sharing of any part of this book without the permission of the publisher is unlawful piracy and theft of the author's intellectual property. If you would like to use material from the book (other than for review purposes), prior written permission must be obtained by contacting GlobalPublishingGroupLLC@gmail.com

This is a work of creative non-fiction. The opinions expressed in this book are those of the authors and not necessarily the views of Global Publishing Group LLC.

Printed in the United States of America

First trade edition: August 2019

ISBN 978-1-6893562-0-6

MEN -TAKE O - PAUSE

DEDICATION

This book is dedicated to every woman who has lived through menopause, is currently in the burning throes of it or who will encounter it at some point in her lifetime.

Remember, you will survive... though I can't promise that to the man in your life.

Hopefully, this book will help him navigate the menopausal darkness and find light at the end of the tunnel. May it not be a train.

Men -Take-O - Pause

INTRODUCTION

I am typically a suspense novelist but delved into this topic in the non-fiction realm because it is near and dear to my heart; and I believe there is a need for it. This book was birthed out of discussions with hundreds of menopausal women and the realization that, despite their varying degrees of symptoms, they all share a common angst. They wish that the men in their lives could understand their menopausal mindset.

As I write this book it is with the intent to give men some valuable information about menopause and a tiny glimpse into what is

MEN – TAKE – O – PAUSE

happening to the menopausal women in their world. If you, men, have insights into her thoughts, fears and struggles then perhaps the menopausal years will be easier on both of you.

Menopause is life-altering for the woman, true, but what often gets overlooked is how puzzling and even scary it can be for men. Most men are quite literally in the dark when it comes to mood swing triggers and bouts of emotion. The abrupt changes in her can often leave him reeling.

Throughout this book, I will be blunt and there will most assuredly be parts that make you a little uncomfortable; but please keep reading. My hope is that by the end you will have gained helpful information and some do's

MEN – TAKE – O – PAUSE

and don'ts to assist you in navigating the menopausal landmines.

May you find a way to calm the menopausal beast within. ~

MEN - TAKE - O - PAUSE

#1

"If you are male, she will undoubtedly resent you during menopause."

Men -Take-O - Pause

CHAPTER ONE

Resentment

We need to start with the basics. You're a man. She's a woman. Her body has most likely gone through more chemical changes throughout her lifetime than yours; from the onset of her period to the histrionic changes during pregnancy and now, menopause. Each change is dramatic in its own way and emotionally symbolizes a stage of life. Her period represents the excitement of embracing womanhood. Pregnancy represents new life and the start of a family. Menopause

MEN -TAKE-O - PAUSE

represents aging and ultimately death. So, you can already see the grim mindset of the menopausal woman.

With this mindset comes a certain resentment that she may not have ever felt nor verbalized before. A subconscious resentment toward men, not just you, but the male gender as a whole.

Menopause is an uncomfortable reminder that life isn't fair because if it were fair then women wouldn't be the only ones to have periods, birth children and experience menopause.

During menopause, she becomes keenly aware that the aging cards are stacked in favor of the male gender. As she gains weight, has hot flashes and feels like she's losing her mind, she sees men coping with mid-life crisis, (the male equivalent of menopause) by dating younger women, getting hair plugs and buying sports cars. The underlying societal meme that men grow distinguished and more respected with age and women get old and discarded, haunts her. With this perspective, you can certainly understand why her injustice meter is spinning.

Resentment is a typical symptom of menopause so try not to take it personally. It isn't your fault. You aren't the Creator who chose to make the female gender endure these chemical changes. Though, He is also a man, which is a fact she may be prone to spew during a resentful rage.

MEN -TAKE- O - PAUSE

During the course of her menopausal years, you will undoubtedly face this unjust resentment. Try to remind yourself in those moments that she is unable to control this feeling, that you have *most likely* done nothing to provoke it, and that it will eventually subside.

Men-take-pause... and breathe. This is only the beginning.

Men-Take-O-Pause

#2

"No man will escape menopause without knowing how little he knows."

CHAPTER TWO

No Escape

The menopausal woman is keenly aware that she has no options. There is no stopping menopause. There is no way around it, no bypass, no alternate route. She's in the tunnel, the train is bearing down and there's nowhere to run. Thus, she feels trapped, stuck, imprisoned in her own body. She longs for the feeling of freedom though she doesn't really know what that means. She's frustrated and afraid.

To add to that plight is the burden of truth that whether your relationship survives or not, she still faces menopause. You can walk away but there is no escape for her. This, in and of itself, is another injustice in her mind.

Medication can often help minimize the hot flashes and ease the highs and lows of the emotional roller coaster, but it can't get her or you off the ride altogether. And unfortunately, medication can't stop the aging process and the symptomatic psychological effects thereof.

She feels old and there's not a pill in the world to take that feeling away.

She's afraid she'll never be perceived as pretty or beautiful again; and no medication can remove that fear.

Men-Take-O-Pause

She despises her body, her weight gain, her lack of flexibility, her low libido. There is no magic pill to fix this.

Knowing these things about her will hopefully help you understand that when she lashes out at you, it is rarely personal. It feels personal because you're the center of her rage; but deep down, you aren't the real problem and she knows it. When she nitpicks at you, it is a mere transference of how she feels about herself. It's her inner child screaming at the injustice that you, the male, don't have to go through any of this. It's her way of stomping her feet and crossing her arms and yelling, "It isn't fair!"

She doesn't hate you, even though she may profess loathing at times. She hates what is happening to her. She doesn't think you're stupid, even though she might call you an idiot at times. It is merely an expression of her frustration over the fact that, as a man, you cannot empathize with her struggle.

The truth is she wants you to understand. She needs you to understand. And the irony is that she knows she's asking the impossible.

There is no escape and this makes daily life a little scary. When she goes to sleep at night, she doesn't know what she's waking up to the next morning; and, truthfully, neither do you.

She needs you to be there in the moments of irrational sadness, even if she strikes out at you. Armor up and be her

MEN -TAKE-O - PAUSE

strength. Because there is no escape, she needs you to be the hero of her heart in her darkest hour. She needs you to battle the beast.

Men-take-pause.

#3

"It is impossible for you to understand what she is feeling so don't try to be empathetic; you need only to become an expert at being sympathetic."

CHAPTER THREE

Don't Tell Her You "Understand"

There are times when a man can utter the phrase, "I understand," and it validates a woman's feelings. An episode of Two and a Half Men comes to mind, where Charlie discovers that uttering the phrase, "I understand" makes women feel heard and understood. By validating their emotions, he finds that they are more prone to trust him and thereby more likely to engage in a sexual relationship. Under normal circumstances, telling a woman that you understand what she

MEN -TAKE-O - PAUSE

is feeling is a good thing; but during menopause it is not.

That phrase doesn't work during menopause because she's not an idiot. She knows the truth and the truth is, you *don't* understand. It's not your fault. It is biologically impossible for you to understand. The only thing you could remotely liken menopause to is pregnancy and you can't understand that either. As a man, you have no life experience in this department so when you utter the phrase, "I understand," what a woman hears is patronizing dribble. Thus, when you say this phrase, she will unjustly and unintentionally view you one of two ways: either lacking the intuition to be able to sympathize with her -or- too arrogant to admit that you don't know what is going on. So, protect yourself because telling her you "understand" will only infuriate her and make her want to hurl heavy objects in your general direction.

The truth is that she knows you don't get it and deep down she doesn't expect you to get it. Most of the time *she* doesn't even know what is happening in her own body or why she feels the way she feels. So, how could you possibly know? She doesn't want you to lie to her and pretend to know how to make it better. *She* doesn't even know how to make it better. She doesn't need you to fix her. She merely needs you to validate her emotions by being intuitive, sympathetic and attentive.

She needs you to be intuitive, sympathetic and attentive.

Most men are spectacular at being helpful when they know what to do. But many men struggle to figure out how to be helpful when they're not given specifics and they have to intuitively figure it out on their own; which, by the way, is exactly what the menopausal woman wants you to do.

She wants you to give her what she needs even when she may or may not know exactly what that is. You see the quandary you are in, right?

So, of course, you do what any man would do and logically attempt to figure out what she needs by applying rational thought to

Men-take-pause

a menopausal-driven emotional problem. And it blows up in your face, leaving you perplexed as to what you did wrong.

Men-take-pause.

You no longer dwell in a reality that is action driven. Things are no longer clear cut. Instead, her perception is the new reality. What she perceives to be your intent behind every action drives her emotional response, regardless of whether it is logical or even accurate.

Her perception is the new reality in which you dwell. It's a reality that is not real to you but very real to her.

I will not lie to you; this new reality is booby trapped. Unfortunately, that doesn't mean there are a lot of boobies. In fact, during menopause, with her radically changing libido, you may feel like you never get to see any boobies at all. We'll address this in a later chapter and hopefully get you to a place where you'll find a *Tit-for-Tat* balance; ultimately giving you more booby time.

Knowing this new reality is booby trapped means you have to tweak your perspective on reality so that you can navigate through the menopausal minefield and avoid future explosions. Remember, *her* perception is the only reality that exists in her menopausal mind.

MEN -TAKE-O - PAUSE

It seems impossible, doesn't it? Don't lose hope. It's true that you may not be able to understand or empathize with what is happening to her, but that doesn't mean you are incapable of helping her through it. And the reality is, even if she doesn't say it, she needs your help now more than ever.

MEN – TAKE – O – PAUSE

#4

"When in doubt, shut the f@#k up."

MEN -TAKE- O - PAUSE

CHAPTER FOUR

Silence is Golden

There is a vast difference between the estrogen-minded woman and the testosterone-minded man. This difference is magnified during menopause, which means, like it or not, you have to watch what you say. If you are a betting man, you can almost take to the bank the fact that what seems like a non-offensive, witty remark will be misunderstood, misinterpreted and result in a fight.

MEN -TAKE-O - PAUSE

So, whenever a snarky comment sneaks into your head, no matter how humorous you think it may be, reach up to your lips and cover them with your palm so it cannot spill out. During menopause, snide remarks could get you killed.

Though there are thousands of things a man should never say to a menopausal woman, I want to give you just a few examples of the most common phrases.

It would behoove you to steer clear of these phrases and anything remotely like them. In fact, if you are not one hundred percent positive that something you are about to say will be well-received, don't speak. Silence is golden and it just might save your life.

MEN -TAKE-O - PAUSE

Avoidable Phrase #1:

"Is it hot in here or is it just you?"

From a male perspective, when you utter this phrase, you think you're being whimsical and witty and trying to lighten the mood. For you it's a nudge-nudge-wink-wink, hardy-har-har kind of moment. For her, it's not. For her it's a stare you down, snarl and envision slapping you, kind of moment. She doesn't think it's funny and here's why:

During a hot flash, the last thing a woman feels is sexy. The last thing on her mind is the thought of appearing attractive or "hot." In fact, she is keenly aware that she's a bloated, sweaty, unfeminine mess. She feels out of control and ugly. The hair that she spent time curling or straightening, is now damp and stuck to her face. The make-up she tediously applied, in what she now sees as a hopeless attempt to look younger and prettier, is smeared by perspiration. She feels wet in every crevice of her body and her sweat smells like a hormonal teenage boy. It dampens her armpits, forms a puddle beneath each breast, and runs down her ass crack. In that moment, she feels disgusting. And worse than that, she feels afraid because she has absolutely no control of what is happening in her body. To her, there is nothing amusing about a hot flash. It is literally the epitome of fear-laced nausea rolled in the stench of death.

So, when you utter that phrase, two things happen: first, she thinks you're being a jerk, rubbing in her face the fact that she is the farthest thing from "hot." Second, it becomes clear in her mind that you have absolutely no idea what she is suffering and that makes her feel very much alone.

She can't see beyond what is happening in her body and mind to realize that you are simply trying to lighten the mood. She won't appreciate the attempt, so protect yourself and refrain from any "hot" jokes.

Avoidable Phrase #2:

"Don't worry about the weight gain, you're still beautiful to me."

Men – Take – O – Pause

Rule of thumb: For your own safety it is best not to utter a sentence to a woman that includes a combination of the words, "weight" and "gain." In any stage of life, this will not bode well for you.

From a male perspective, when you say this sentence, you think you're saying something sweet and soothing, something to make her feel secure. After all, how could telling a woman that you will always find her beautiful be a bad thing? Hide and watch.

You think you're calling her beautiful and professing the unconditional depth of your love. But you're not. Not even close. What that sentence is *really* doing is implying that she is no longer beautiful to the rest of the world and boasting that, despite her weight

Men -JAKE- O - Pause

gain and eluded to lack of beauty, you have the strength to still love her. You're flattering yourself, not her. You're calling her fat and then offering pity masked as affection. It's a terribly hurtful statement and if you're dumb enough to utter it...RUN!

Avoidable Phrase #3"

"Why are you so bitchy?"

If a man said this to me, my response would be, "Why are you such an asshole?" Which will probably be exactly what she's thinking. So, despite the fact that there may be factual evidence to support that she is being "bitchy," don't say it. It will not end well for you.

The short answer to the question, "Why is she so bitchy?" is that her whole body is changing and she has no control over any of it. She is uncomfortable and out-of-place in her own skin. She is fearful and frustrated.

The long answer is that lasting bitchiness ultimately comes from her perception that her needs are not being met.

Lasting bitchiness may be derived from remarks she deemed hurtful or moments when she felt ignored or misunderstood. Bitchiness can very well stem from the feeling that she is utterly alone.

MEN –TAKE O – PAUSE

Before your defenses flare and you think I'm saying that her bitchiness is all *your* fault, let me explain. It's not all your fault, nor is it all her fault. It is simply and unfortunately a menopausal reality due to the changes in her body and mind.

For a menopausal woman, the buffer in her brain that normally exists, is suddenly gone. That buffer allowed her to breeze over your remarks or poorly timed jokes and still see you as cute. It allowed her to give you credit for trying, even if you fell short. The buffer allowed her to see your intent and not just your actions.

During menopause, that buffer dissipates and she suddenly discovers the unsettling reality that you might not know her as well as she thought you did. She begins to re-analyze everything you've ever done and said. Suddenly, without the buffer, she is no longer able to NOT notice your shortcomings. They are highlighted in her brain.

And it gets worse. Though she loves you, all of a sudden and simultaneously, there are moments when she finds herself barely able to stand you. This is no fault of your own. It is simply a change in her chemistry. Loving and loathing now share a space in her head and which one takes top billing and thereby controls her mood depends highly on her perception of whether or not her needs are being met.

This often gets confusing for men because you are biologically designed to meet

MEN-TAKE-O-PAUSE

the physical and practical needs of the woman you love. You are a provider and you've probably been good at it thus far. You've probably been adequately meeting her needs for years. All of sudden, the bar is raised and you're expected to meet her emotional needs that have no clear-cut definition. They are vague at best.

Without warning, her brain is demanding justice and validation. She wants affection in ways that are foreign to your thinking. She's dishing out ultimatums and making demands that she has never made before. Her motto has clearly become, "My way or the highway," and you're a little more than shaken by the dramatic changes in her.

Men-take-pause.

MEN –TAKE–O – PAUSE

The menopausal mindset is done paying it forward. She wants what she believes she deserves and she wants to be loved in the manner in which her heart now requires. There are no more ifs-ands-buts or in-betweens; and she accepts no more excuses. She will resent you if her needs are not being met and blame you for it; which will make her "bitchy" toward you.

The good news is eventually her chemistry will rebalance and the buffer will reappear. The bad news is it won't be too soon. So, if you decide to bring her bitchiness to her attention, you best be ready to duck and cover.

MEN -TAKE- O - PAUSE

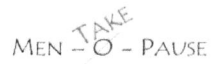

Avoidable Phrase #4:

"How long is this menopause thing going to last?"

This phrase is another big no-no. You might think you're asking a valid question, seeking information as one might in a typical medical situation. For example, after a surgical procedure one might ask the doctor, "How long after surgery will it take for me to return to normal?" It seems like a fine, logical question. But, with regards to menopause, it is not. It's a very, very bad question and you should never ask it to a menopausal woman.

Despite how the question is phrased, what you're *really* asking and what she hears you asking is *how long do you have to put up with her. How long do you have to tolerate her?* What you are really telling her with this question is that you don't like her this way and you want her to change back. Her deeper perception of this question is that you can't handle what's happening and that you're not in this together. This causes her to feel alone and vulnerable. What's worse is that this simple question has now made her doubt your strength and fear the eventual dissolution of your relationship.

When you ask this question, she sees that you are obviously tolerating her presence, which makes her feel unloved. This grows insecurity and fear in her heart. It also produces anger and more resentment toward you.

You must keep in mind that she didn't do anything to cause this biological change in her. Time did. Age did. She is powerless to alter the course and change back. If she could, she would. So, when you ask this question, she feels like you are blaming her for something over which she has absolutely no control.

Statistically, the average length of menopause is four years, though some women experience symptoms much longer, lasting from seven to twelve years. Every woman's body is unique so it's difficult to pinpoint an exact amount of time. Of one thing you can be certain, menopause lasts longer than either of you desire.

MEN - JAKE O - PAUSE

Avoidable Phrase #5:

"Calm down."

To you, this is a logical statement. To her, it's a catalyst for violence and/or tears.

You've probably already noticed that a menopausal woman, whose buffer is gone, is prone to ranting. Her ranting can undoubtedly become tiresome for you. Honestly, it's exhausting for her, as well, but if she doesn't rant her frustrations her head is likely to explode.

When you tell a menopausal woman to "calm down" it is the equivalent of throwing gasoline on a fire. The moment that phrase leaves your lips and hits her ears, she loathes

MEN -TAKE-O - PAUSE

you. She genuinely in her core, from the tippy top of her sweaty head down to the very point of her big toe, can't stand you.

Why? How can one tiny statement cause love and loathing to collide in her brain and make her want to throw things at you?

First, she doesn't believe you, or anyone for that matter, has the right to tell her to calm down. Her emotions are raw and real and raging and it is not possible for her to embrace calm. The fact that you try to apply logic to this emotion only makes her feel all the more that you do not understand her or what is happening in her body. Telling her to calm down is basically telling her that she is alone on an island, that you'll never understand her, and you'll never get it.

Second, when you tell her to calm down, she will feel as though you are being condescending. You may simply be trying to soothe what is happening in the moment, but she will not see it that way. Remember, *her* perception is the new reality in which you both dwell.

When you tell her to calm down, she will think that you deem her emotional rage a weakness. She will think that because you appear in control of your faculties, you're belittling her for not being in control of hers. Even if a condescending tone is far from your intent, she will see it as prevalent in your approach and blame you for it anyway.

Remember, you're dealing with hormone-driven emotion, not rational thinking. It doesn't have to be fair and it rarely will be.

A fact you need to face is that if you make the mistake of telling her to calm down, you then become the catalyst for escalating her rage. That falls on you. So, protect yourself and don't do it.

Men-take-pause. Understand that the male ego has no place in menopause. What I mean by that is that if she senses any form of arrogance, her defenses will rise. The menopausal beast is locked and loaded and will shoot arrogance down on sight. Thus, your approach to her has to be altered so that she cannot misinterpret your words.

So, what can you do to calm her down when she is upset?

MEN -TAKE-O - PAUSE

When she rants, let her. Don't mock. Don't mimic. Don't defend the other party. Don't point out another perspective. For God's sake, don't roll your eyes. Don't exhale loudly to denote that you are tired of hearing her speak. Don't shake your head in disagreement or disgust. Don't leave the room as if you cannot stand to be around her when she's ranting. This will make her even more resentful.

Instead, sit quietly, giving her your full attention and nodding every so often until the rage subsides. Then, simply wrap your arms around her sweaty torso and tell her that you love her. This is your only hope for survival because if you tell her to calm down you will become the focus of her rage.

MEN -TAKE O - PAUSE

Avoidable Phrase #6:

"You're getting upset over nothing."

This is yet another phrase I would not recommend uttering to a woman at any stage of life, but in menopause it will generate one of two reactions. Either she will burst into tears or she will pick up the nearest object and try to bludgeon you with it.

When you tell a woman that she is "getting upset over nothing" you are invalidating everything she feels. In essence, you are telling her that her feelings are irrelevant. Meaningless. Ridiculous. Not real and not worth discussing. This is not only incredibly hurtful but produces fierce amounts

MEN -TAKE-O- PAUSE

of anger. Anger that will undeniably resurface with every argument you have going forward.

What you're really trying to say with that statement is that you don't understand why she is getting so upset; but that isn't the message conveyed with those words.

Instead of thinking you are trying to understand her, she will feel as though you are belittling her feelings and therefore will offer you no respect in return. Even if you were not intentionally trying to be aloof, the moment this phrase leaves your lips, she will view you as a cold-hearted prick. I warned you in the beginning of this book that I would be blunt. I use this verbiage intentionally to drive home the point that the menopausal woman's mindset encases the extremes and radically

MEN-TAKE-O-PAUSE

bounces between them. She is literally incapable of giving you the benefit of the doubt. Thus, in any given situation you are either a wonderful man or a cold-hearted prick. There is little option in-between. So, if you don't want to be seen as the cold-hearted prick, choose your words carefully and don't utter phrases that can be construed as aloof or non-sympathetic.

There are a million examples of phrases you should not verbalize in her menopausal presence. To be safe, you need to consume a daily, heaping helping of common sense and intuition before you speak. When in doubt, remind yourself that silence is golden and shut up.

MEN -TAKE-O - PAUSE

You might be thinking that this isn't fair. Why should you conform your thoughts, words and opinions to behavior you deem irrational? Why does she have license to say anything she wants and you can't? Why does she get to have all of the control?

For some men, dwelling in her perception of things feels emasculating. But allow me to tweak that perspective.

She knows that only the strongest of men are able to set their ego aside in order to love a woman in the manner in which she needs to be loved... especially when the circumstances aren't fair. She knows that only men of great stability and mental fortitude are capable of sacrificing their opinion for the woman they love, and she sees this as a gesture of strength, not weakness. This is not about winning or getting the last word. This is about loving deeply and making sacrifices when necessary to show that love.

We've all heard the saying, "Love conquers all," which comes from I Corinthians in the Bible. With regards to menopause, love conquers the menopausal monster by disarming it.

To disarm it, you must first understand what triggers the beast to draw its weapons. The menopausal beast rears its ugly head when a woman feels unloved, unnoticed or not understood. So, to battle the hormone-driven mindset with rational, ego-driven force will only make defenses rise and result in arguments, resentment and hurt feelings.

MEN – TAKE – O – PAUSE

When both of you are heated, neither of you feels in control of what is happening and the menopausal beast wins. This isn't good for anyone.

The only way to control the beast is by relinquishing control, which in a twist of irony gives you exactly what you want... to avoid a fight, minimize conflict and have peace in your home. When you sacrifice your need to be right in order to save the relationship, you are not weak in her eyes; but stronger than you have ever been before. That's how you win.

To quiet the beast, one must love quietly even when the circumstances aren't fair.

Men-take-pause.

#5

"The menopausal beast is real. Don't underestimate its power."

Men –TAKE–O– Pause

CHAPTER FIVE

It's All in Her Head

It is frightening to learn that there are actually men who believe that menopause is all in a woman's head, and if that woman would conquer such irrational thoughts, she would remain stable and otherwise "normal." These men are idiots. They should have their mouths permanently sewn shut for the duration of menopause. Thankfully, they do not represent the majority of the male population.

Menopause is a mental, emotional and chemical alteration of the female body, one

Men -TAKE-O - Pause

over which she has no control. Her hormone levels change and even with medication women can't always find balance. Every day is like riding a roller coaster in the dark with no safety harness. She can't see the track. She doesn't know where she's heading. She's simply hanging on for dear life and praying it will be over soon.

There are plenty of physical symptoms offering validation that menopause is far from something women have contrived in their minds. But I think part of the challenge for men is that they can't see what is happening inside of a woman. They can't feel the changes like she can so they are often caught off guard by the manifestations of those changes. Men see the mood swing but they are unable to see

Men -Take- O - Pause

the trigger. Thus, they unknowingly stumble into the beast's booby traps.

To help you better understand what can be perceived as erratic irritability, here are just a few of the things happening to a woman's body during menopause:

- ✓ She wakes up soaked in the middle of the night from horrendous night sweats that then leave her shivering and cold from being wet. She's literally wet from the back of her neck to the back of her knees. Sometimes she's so wet that she wonders if she has peed in the bed. She gets up, showers and changes into a clean pair of pajamas, crawls back into bed and hopes it doesn't happen again.

You sleep through it, which she finds irritating and unfair.

✓ She suffers from insomnia and hence exhaustion. And at 3:00am when she glances over at you sleeping like a baby, she wants to strangle you.

✓ She gets hormonal headaches that Ibuprofen and Tylenol can't touch, and yet she functions through them because she has no other choice. But the constant ache adds to her irritability.

✓ Her breasts swell and ache at any given moment with absolutely no warning. Thus, when you come up behind her

Men –TAKE–O– Pause

and grab them, thinking you're being affectionate, it causes pain and pisses her off.

- ✓ She feels famished even when she's just eaten and she craves food at odd hours. When you make comments like, "How can you be hungry? We just ate!" This makes her feel fat, makes her believe that you think she's fat and thereby causes her to feel guilty about desiring food. It also makes her angry and she may envision beating you over the head with a large hoagie.

MEN -JAKE O - PAUSE

✓ She feels like she's pregnant but there is no baby, no extra attention, no sympathy, no glowing and no reward.

✓ She gains weight in places that she didn't use to gain weight. Women often get pudgy tummies, expansive hips, flabby thighs and back fat during menopause. No matter what she does, the weight doesn't easily come off. This causes her to feel unattractive and frustrated because some of her favorite outfits no longer fit. It also intensifies her fear that you will stop being attracted to her and ultimately stop loving her.

MEN -TAKE-O - PAUSE

- ✓ She feels ugly, sweaty and unfeminine most of the time and her self-esteem takes a dive.

- ✓ She cries when she looks in the mirror.

- ✓ She realizes that she's aging and she fears that beauty is slipping away. She's afraid to grow old. She's afraid of what it means to grow old. All she sees are the things over which she has no control and she feels an overwhelming sense of doom and pending death.

- ✓ She becomes keenly aware that according to societal standards you grow "distinguished" while she grows "old." She subconsciously resents you for this.

✓ She feels insecure about your relationship and fears you will trade her in for a younger version. This fear prompts feelings of worry, jealousy and distrust.

✓ There are mornings when she wakes up feeling sad and doesn't know why. This sadness can linger throughout the day and she has to fight to hide the tears from those around her. This makes her feel raw and emotionally unraveled as she tries not to succumb to full-blown depression. She feels ashamed and quietly berates herself for not being strong enough to handle it.

- ✓ Her buffer is gone and she suddenly sees the world as a place filled with stupid people making stupid mistakes. She hates these people and is aware that she has become less tolerant of others and what she sees as their perpetual bullshit. This makes her want to hide away from the world and so she isolates herself, thereby increasing her loneliness.

- ✓ Her periods become erratic and come and go without warning, further limiting her wardrobe options and often intensifying her bloating and discomfort.

- ✓ Things that used to make her feel good, like massages or lying in a tanning bed now feel uncomfortable and can cause a certain sense of panic.

- ✓ Physical touch that used to stimulate her now feels disconnected and bothersome.

- ✓ Her sex drive plummets and becomes almost non-existent. She feels guilty about this and at the same time, irritated that, despite everything going on in her body, there is the unspoken and/or often verbalized expectation that she still owes you sex. She begins to resent this expectation, resent you because of it and sex becomes just one more item on her to-do list.

✓ She is prone to greater mood swings than she's ever experienced before and she feels out of control.

✓ She begins to question everything about life, spirituality and death. She feels like a timer is ticking faster and faster and she's running out of time. She wonders if she had made all of the wrong decisions and wasted her one chance at living.

Men –TAKE– O – Pause

- ✓ She feels afraid to die.

- ✓ Her taste buds have suddenly changed and foods and drinks that she used to love have become flavorless or distasteful.

- ✓ Her sense of smell is magnified so the slightest odor can repel her and make her instantly irritable. Without her buffer she is prone to loudly announce that someone in the room stinks!

- ✓ She has hot flashes during the day that render her on the verge of passing out or throwing up and cause her to strip down to her underwear and shove herself into the freezer. Sometimes a

MEN -TAKE-O - PAUSE

hot flash can be so strong that she fears she is having a heart attack and that she's going to die.

✓ She can't remember things, like simple, basic words and she begins to doubt her sanity and reliability and/or fear she is suffering from early onset Alzheimer's.

✓ She has trouble concentrating and often feels overwhelmed by loud noises and simultaneous conversations.

✓ Her bladder isn't what it used to be and she is keenly aware that a big sneeze or a bout of laughter can cause her to piddle in her panties.

✓ Her skin and hair have changed, becoming brittle and dry, making her alter her routines and products in an attempt to find normalcy again.

✓ There is suddenly less vaginal lubrication, which can make penetration feel like someone is rubbing sandpaper on her cooter. Thus, when she perceives that you have an expectation of her to continue to sexually satisfy you regardless of how she is feeling, she becomes embittered.

These are but a few general examples. As I previously mentioned, menopause is unique to each woman so symptoms can vary from non-existent to unbearable. With all of this going on in her body and mind, the last thing she needs is a man condescendingly asking her how long this menopause thing is going to last or telling her what a tribulation it is for *him*. Can you see how an attitude like that might infuriate her?

Believe me, she knows it's no walk in the park for you. She knows this to such degree that she wrestles with feelings of guilt. At the same time, she cannot belay the expectations of her heart.

The menopausal woman expects her husband to strap himself into the roller coaster next to her, hold her hand and shut up. She doesn't expect him to have any answers or to be able to fix her. But she does expect him to realize that this is about *her*, not about him and refrain from pointing out how difficult or inconvenient menopause is for *him*. She will be incapable of offering him empathy unless she first feels an outpouring of his sympathy.

Her world is changing, as is her perception of reality. You are living in her reality now and though it may not be fair, logical or comfortable, you must learn to exist in it in order to survive menopause.

Men-take-pause.

#6

"Menopausal women do not nag. They make suggestions. Vigorously."

CHAPTER SIX
Nag. Nag. Nag.

If you're wondering why all of a sudden it seems that the woman in your life is riding your ass about EVERYTHING and you can't do anything right, welcome to menopause. Now is the time for you, men, to take pause. Now is the time for you to reassess everything you thought you knew about her, because chances are it's all changing.

The simple fact is that she barely knows herself anymore which means there's no possible way you can know her.

Everything about her world is a bubble off plum now. It's ever so slightly tweaked. Everything of which she thought she was certain is now laced with uncertainty. Things that worked for her and satisfied her before don't anymore. She doesn't know why, so don't bother asking her.

She wants things to be different because she wants desperately to feel better...better about herself, better about you, better about life. The problem is she doesn't know how to get there and can't really even define what "better" means.

It is not uncommon to see the menopausal woman alter exterior things in a subconscious attempt to fix the interior. She might buy a new car, open her own credit card accounts, change her name, opt for a new hairstyle or dye her hair a new color. She might take off on a road trip by herself, get a tattoo or body piercing, change churches or stop going to church altogether. She might begin to hate TV shows she once loved and love shows she swore she'd never watch. She might completely alter her wardrobe and her style or buy new furniture, curtains, carpet, dishes, etc. These things and more are merely outward grasps to gain control of what is happening inside her body, mind and soul.

Where does that leave you? Trying desperately to keep up.

The best thing you can do is face the fact that right now you know nothing about her. But, don't let this get you down. Instead, look at it as a challenge. Do you have what it takes to re-learn everything about her? Are you strong enough to walk with her through the darkness? Do you have the stamina for the long-haul? Can you prove it, because, if you want the nagging to stop, you're going to have to prove it.

As I mentioned in a previous chapter, the buffer in her that used to tolerate your flaws and give you credit for attempted goodness, is now gone. Menopause has raised the bar and what this means for you is that you're going to have to bring your A-game.

I know it doesn't sound fair, but you have to keep in mind that what's happening to her isn't "fair" either. She has no control over the changes occurring in her body. Try to remember that as uncomfortable as all of this makes you, it is affecting her ten times more.

As best as you can, try to remind yourself that this is about *her*, not you. The simple fact is that as she changes, you must alter your approach to her, like it or not, fair or not. If you want your relationship to survive, you're going to have to be willing to make changes.

Menopause has removed her ability to see beyond your flaws. Not just your flaws, but the whole world's flaws. Believe me, nobody is getting off easy in her eyes. She's looking at the world though a menopausal microscope that renders it impossible for her to ignore something that bothers her. Everything that bothers her is magnified. Since

Men – Take – O – Pause

you're the person who probably spends the most time with her, it stands to reason that your habits, quirks and idiosyncrasies are going to be forefront in the line of fire. Whether it's the way you chew your food, put on your shoes or simply the sound of your voice, she's suddenly tired of all of it. She wants change.

So, are you supposed to walk on egg shells for several years? No. My recommendation is that you walk around the egg shells, because if you step on one, you're going to hear about it.

Seriously, though, your job is to navigate through the menopausal landmines and you do this by proactively paying attention to every little detail. In short, if you want the complaining to stop, you've got to stop giving her reasons to complain. This is where the rubber meets the road and every expression of your love must bear the burden of proof.

Is it fair that your every move is being scrutinized by the menopausal beast within? No. But the irony lies in the fact that to calm the beast you must examine *her* every move. You must know her thoroughly in order to proactively meet her needs; and when those needs are met, the scrutinizing of you stops.

In short, knowledge is power and your key to a nag-free existence.

Let me give you an example. Let's say you come home with what you think is her favorite box of chocolate. You don't have a clue that it isn't her favorite anymore. So, while you think you're doing something good and romantic, all she sees is the fact that you don't *really know her.* Because if you really knew her, you'd have known that this wasn't her favorite chocolate anymore. Instead of making her feel loved, you have inadvertently made her feel alone and unnoticed. With her buffer no longer in-tact, this action is considered a fail and you get no credit for the chocolate nor the thought behind it.

I can almost feel your jaws dropping at the insensitive injustice of what I've just told you. But bear with me boys, as we dive even deeper into the female menopausal psyche.

The pre-menopausal-her would have given you credit for thinking of her and buying the chocolate in the first place, even if it wasn't her favorite. In fact, the pre-menopausal-her would have let you believe that it was her favorite and that you had successfully shown your love through this romantic gesture. The pre-menopausal-her would have applauded your efforts.

But the pre-menopausal-her is dead. She's gone. Her brain is no longer the same. It has been chemically altered. Let her go. The sooner you accept this fact, the better chance you have of survival.

The menopausal-her needs ongoing proof that she is known, noticed and valued.

That proof comes from you being perfect in every word and gesture. This means you have to pay attention… to everything.

The tiniest things can often matter the most. Showing up with the wrong chocolate, as trivial and ridiculous as it sounds, can result in an argument that lasts for days and hurt feelings that never go away.

The little things can either make her feel incredibly loved or painfully unnoticed. Remember, the menopausal mindset lives in the extremes, not in the in-between. She feels quite literally either loved or hated. The gray area, the buffer zone, is gone. So, the tiniest gestures can either make or break her heart. You have to be able to decipher which is which without her telling you ahead of time. This is no easy task and undoubtedly makes you feel like you are tip toeing through a minefield. In essence, you are.

Everyone has a basic human need to feel that they are known and loved by another person. There's something soothing about looking across the room at your spouse and smiling because each of you knows what the other is thinking. There's a sense of security and safety in being known and in the acceptance that comes with it.

For the menopausal woman, being known now equates to being loved.

I'm going to repeat that one more time because it is the crux of the menopausal mindset and at the driving core of all of her emotions. *For the menopausal woman, being known now equates to being loved.*

For her, everything is changing and she barely recognizes herself. With this, births a deep-rooted fear that you will cease to recognize her. Remember, this fear isn't rational, it's emotional and extremely powerful. Thus, when she has to tell you how to love her, she feels unknown; and that unknown sensation makes her feel unloved and lost.

Take that information back to the chocolate example: If she has to tell you what her favorite kind of chocolate is then she is forced to face the realization that you don't know. In her mindset there exists only one possible reason why you don't know: you don't love her enough to pay attention. This makes her feel unnoticed and alone.

Men –TAKE O – Pause

The menopausal woman needs you to intuitively recognize her needs and then proactively meet them without her uttering a word.

To the male, rational, logical mindset, this sounds ludicrous. You must shake your head and think I'm asking the impossible. You're right. It is impossible... that is, if you attempt it from a rational, logical mindset. But there is another way.

I won't lie and tell you it's easy, but it is doable. And when you do it, you will make her feel known, noticed and valued. You will make her realize that she is not alone. You will show her that she is deeply loved. This is when the nagging stops.

This will require all of your attention and more emotional effort than you've probably had to put into the relationship in a long time. The reality of marriage is that over time we settle into a comfort zone. When we've been together a long time, we stop working hard at the relationship and just sort-of exist within it.

Menopause is rattling the comfort zone and shaking up that existence.

You're still the same you but she's no longer the same her.

This forces you to adapt to the new reality and get to know her all over again. In this get-to-know-her-again process, there are some pitfalls you should try to avoid.

Pitfall #1: Never Make Assumptions

Never make assumptions. Keep in mind that she is changing, sometimes week to week, sometimes day to day, sometimes minute to minute. For you to assume anything could be deadly.

This brings to memory a personal example, one in which I look back on and laugh; but it wasn't funny at the time. I was at the beginning of my menopausal years, and one night my husband decided he would order pizza for our family. He was doing something nice by lightening my load so I didn't have to

MEN -JAKE- O - PAUSE

worry about cooking dinner that night. He ordered what we always ordered: pepperoni and sausage pizza. All of a sudden, I was consumed with a sense of injustice and anger. I exploded into a rant about how I had been eating *his* favorite pizza for twenty years and he had never even once bothered to ask what *my* favorite pizza was. He stood wide-eyed, a deer in headlights, dumbfounded by my reaction. I had never reacted this way to ordering pizza. In fact, I had always been grateful and excited to order pizza.

Finally, when I had stopped my verbal vomit, he uttered cautiously, "What's your favorite pizza?"

"Supreme!" I shrieked. "I like supreme pizza! If you knew me at all you'd know this. I

Men –TAKE–O– Pause

like black olives and onions and green peppers and mushrooms!"

He had no idea because for the first twenty years of our marriage eating pepperoni and sausage pizza didn't bother me. I liked it well enough, even though it wasn't my absolute favorite. I had never said anything about it... until menopause dissipated my buffer and the injustice of twenty years of eating pepperoni and sausage pizza consumed me. I blamed the poor guy for twenty years of what I now deemed as selfish pizza ordering.

Do you see how irrational and spontaneous the menopausal mindset can be?

I share that story to say this, during menopause expect the unexpected and never assume anything.

For example, if your wife has had a glass of red wine every night for the past twenty-five years, should you assume she wants red wine tonight? NO! You should never assume anything. Just because she used to like something or used to do something doesn't mean she likes it or wants to do it anymore. You're living day to day now. Everything you knew about her is void. *Fuhgeddaboudit.*

Confidently assuming you know something can get you into trouble. Here's the rub: *At the same time that you're feeling as if you know nothing about her, you have to make her feel known.*

You're probably thinking, "How the hell do I do that?" It's a good question because, let's face it, you're in quite the predicament.

Let's say you assume, based on her history, that she wants a glass of red wine and you pour the glass and bring it to her. Instead of a gracious thank you, you're met with a narrowed brow and antagonistic glare. You start to backtrack and try to justify why you brought her red wine. But anything you say makes her feel unknown and unnoticed. You have lost this battle before it began.

Instead, tweak your method, thereby protecting yourself and her from an argument. Don't pour her a glass of red wine, but go to her and say something like this, "I know we have red wine most nights, but I was wondering if you might like something different tonight. What would you like?"

If you say that phrase, you're safe. So, memorize it if you need to.

Why does that phrase work? Because as we look deep into the female menopausal psyche, what that phrase has subconsciously told her is that you recognize the changes happening inside of her, that she's not alone in them and that you are willing and able to roll with those changes. This is a huge win for you.

In short, if you want the nagging to stop then you have to stop saying and doing the "wrong" things and start proactively saying and doing the "right" things. How do you know what determines wrong from right? You have to define that on the daily and sometimes minute-by-minute basis by observing and listening to her. This requires all of your conscious attention and emotional effort.

As a rule of thumb in determining how her menopausal mindset labels right from wrong, "wrong" things will generate an angry, hurt or resentful response. "Right" things will generate a sense of calm. Take notes.

Pitfall #2: Don't Apply Logic to Her Emotions

Logic will not apply to most menopausal circumstances and will only cause dissention. You need to understand that her emotional perspective is real to her and validate it as such; even if it isn't necessarily real to you.

What she's feeling doesn't have to make sense to you, and it probably won't much of the time. All you need to do is recognize that it makes sense to her, not try to convince her otherwise.

Your job is not to fix her;
it is to validate her.

But remember, you cannot validate her by uttering a trite, "I understand," because she knows you cannot understand menopause and will think you are being dishonest and patronizing her if you say you do.

What the menopausal woman needs is your patience and support. She needs to feel that you are not only her husband, but also her best friend, who knows her, has her back and is always on her side. This means that often times you will need to keep your opinion to yourself.

In the throes of menopause, what matters more than what you think is that you understand what she thinks.

Again, she knows you cannot understand nor empathize with what is happening in her body. What she needs is to have you understand what is happening in her mind. When you prove that you understand her mindset, she feels safe and accepted. This doesn't mean you have to agree with her thoughts, but rather acknowledge her thinking process.

MEN - TAKE - O - PAUSE

Remember, you can't understand her hormone-driven thought process by applying logic to emotion. Thus, your fact-based opinion doesn't matter. Evidence doesn't matter.

Let me give you an example. If she looks upward and tells you that the sky is purple, and you argue that it is blue, it doesn't matter that you are correct nor that your statement is accurate. You have made her feel disconnected and unknown. But if she says the sky is purple and you respond with, "And a lovely shade of purple it is," you have now made her feel known and accepted. She knows you see blue, but the fact that you are willing to accept that she sees purple is a testament to your love for her. Remember, *in the menopausal mindset being known now equates to being loved.*

That is, of course, an unrealistic example because chances are you both see the sky as blue. However, I use it to paint the picture that if your opinion will make her feel isolated from you instead of connected to you, then perhaps the most loving choice is to keep it to yourself.

Pitfall #3: Never Debate with Her

Never debate with a menopausal woman, even if you know that you are right and her stance on the subject matter is wrong. Even if you have factual and statistical evidence to back up your point, don't do it. You will lose and you'll cause more damage in trying to prove you're right than if you just shut up and let her think that you're on the same page.

The important thing is not about you being right (even if you are right), it's about her feeling connected to you.

This means that there will be times when you will have to make the tough choice to put your ego aside and put her first simply to make her feel loved. This requires sacrifice on your part and can be a very difficult step for some men. It can feel initially emasculating, but if you look through her eyes you will see that when a man lays down his pride for the woman he loves, it is a sign of strength, not weakness. It is in essence you protecting her *even from herself* and it garners her trust, respect and admiration.

Menopause isn't a walk in the park for anyone. It isn't "fair" to anyone. It can be both dangerous and deadly to marriages. Every time you think you can't take one more complaint or nagging comment, try to remember that she isn't enjoying this either. This isn't fun for her. She doesn't want to be the nagging menopausal beast, but more times than not, she can't control the beast. So, as best as you can, try not to give the menopausal monster cause to rear its ugly head.

This is where you, men, must often decide to take one for the team and swallow your pride in the moment...not because you are lessor but because you are making a choice to be greater than the beast.

MEN – TAKE / O – PAUSE

#7

"Put your poker away."

MEN – TAKE – O – PAUSE

CHAPTER SEVEN

Don't Poke the Beast

I'm not going to skirt around nor sugar coat this topic because it's simple and straightforward. Don't poke the beast by poking another woman.

During the menopausal years, everything is heightened. Thus, this is not the time to have an affair. Research has shown that a sexual encounter with another person is ninety-two percent (92%) more likely to end your marriage during menopause than any other time period. Even if your marriage has survived prior

MEN -TAKE-O - PAUSE

indiscretions, chances are, it will not survive infidelity during menopause. So, put your poker away.

One of the greatest challenges during menopause is maintaining a healthy sex life. Statistically speaking, most women experience low-libido during the menopausal years and sexual desire literally falls off her radar. Some women even experience pain during intercourse which makes them further adverse to being intimate. Her low-libido can cause a lack of sexual intimacy in the marriage, often leaving the husband dissatisfied and frustrated.

This, coupled with her severe mood swings, will cause some men to seek sexual satisfaction outside of the marriage. Men will go to strip clubs, pay for lap dances, dive into

MEN -TAKE- O - PAUSE

pornography, engage is meaningless affairs and even hire prostitutes to meet the sexual needs their wife is no longer able to meet.

Some men don't perceive these actions as adulterous because they still love their wife and have no feelings invested in another woman. They don't want a divorce or to start life over with someone new. They simply want sex. Now, let's define sex so we can officially close any and all loopholes. Just so we're clear, we're not using the Bill Clinton definition of sex. Sex is defined as any sexual act, not just intercourse. If you put your poker in another woman's mouth, it's sex. If you put your poker between another woman's breasts, it's sex. If you put your poker in another woman's anus, it's sex. If you put your poker anywhere other than your own hand, it's sex. If you take your poker out in the presence of any woman other than your wife, it's sex. Just because you may not have feelings invested in another woman, doesn't mean your actions aren't adulterous. This is infidelity and your wife will view it as such. So, let me reiterate... put your poker away.

To better understand let's put the shoe on the other foot. At some point the aging process can also negatively affect the male body, making him no longer able to sexually perform the way he could when he was younger. Imagine how you would feel if your wife sought sexual gratification elsewhere because you couldn't satisfy her in bed? Imagine the anger and grief this would bring you. Imagine how crushed you would feel if she gave herself to another man while you were in the stage of life when you were doubting your own manhood. How devastating would this be?

Now that you know that an affair that occurs during the menopausal years is ninety-two percent (92%) more likely to result in divorce than any other time during the marriage, I don't think you want to gamble with those odds. In addition, sixty-three percent (63%) of people engaging in an extra-marital affair eventually get caught. So, the cards are stacked against you and the stakes are higher than they would be during any other stage of life.

You see, the menopausal woman is not equipped to be able to offer take-backs and do-overs. What that means is, she won't be able to forgive you...at least not during menopause.

The menopausal woman is not capable of forgiving something that she deems an intentional act of hatred against her, particularly at her lowest time. Just so we're clear, menopause *is* her lowest time. When you choose to go outside the marriage for sex at a time when she is struggling to get her own body to sexually function, it is not viewed as a "mistake" on your part, but rather an intentional act of hatred against her.

Let me paint a more vivid picture for you. She wouldn't see your infidelity as an

Men -JAKE-O- Pause

"oops, I didn't mean to kick you while you were down" error in judgment. It would be akin to you slamming her to the ground, punching her in the gut, kicking her in the face until she spit up blood in a deliberate act to inflict pain. It would show double the heartlessness, triple the selfishness and quadruple the purposeful intent to cause damage than it would during any other time period. Just as it would for you if the roles were reversed. Outside of a miracle, your marriage will not survive it.

That is a graphic image but hopefully it helps you see what you are doing to her when you seek sexual fulfillment outside of the marriage. You are punishing her for something she can't control. And that is wrong.

Men -Take-O - Pause

Just as you would not get over it, neither will she. Just as you could not grow past it, neither will she. And despite whether you are a good man in every other area of your life, she will view you only as a cold, cruel man and will, at that time and thereafter, want nothing more from you but financial stability. All past goodness will fade and she will see only the infidelity and the fact that you punished her for something out of her control.

To put it more simply, you getting hard for someone else will result in her heart hardening toward you; and you will lose her.

So, put your poker away.

You must understand that everything in the menopausal mindset is magnified and heightened. Thus, is pain and heartache. She is at her worst and she cannot hide it from you. She needs your help and support. She needs to know that you are strong enough to walk with her through the confusion, frustration and dissatisfaction of her low libido. She needs to know that together you can find a road back to sexual intimacy, because even though it might not show, she misses the connection intimacy brings. She misses *you* and your touch.

Right now, her body is working against her and so is her mind. Self-deprecating thoughts hinder her desire for intimacy. When she feels ugly and bloated, tired and sweaty and sick, there is no room for thoughts of sexy and pretty and alluring and close. When she can't stand the way she looks or feels, how can she confidently offer herself to you?

MEN -TAKE-O - PAUSE

Knowing you turned to another woman, while she was at her worst, would destroy her heart and her feelings for you would be incinerated in the flames of your infidelity.

No five-minute fuck is worth the years of agony it will cost you. A lay, no matter how good, is not worth making the woman you love detest you for the rest of your life. And, she would detest you. She wouldn't be able to control the rage that stemmed from the brokenness of your betrayal.

Don't poke the beast.

Don't put your sexual needs above her heart and your marriage. Don't be that selfish when you possess the power to be selfless.

Men -Take-O - Pause

Put your poker away and wait this out with the woman who has earned and deserves your loyalty. Be her hero.

Remember, menopause is temporary. Her libido will jump start again and don't you want to be the man she jumps when it does?

#8

"Menopause in progress... move quietly and do not make eye contact."

MEN -TAKE-O - PAUSE

CHAPTER EIGHT

Back to the Basics

Menopause forces a woman to change, therefore, the man in her life must also change. It's not a "she needs to get through this" problem, it's a "how do WE live through this" issue.

Some days seem impossible. She nitpicks and complains, because to her nothing feels right. You exhale loudly, making your frustration known. She can tell you don't want to be around her. You can tell she doesn't like you. You both wonder why the hell you're still

MEN-TAKE-PAUSE

together. She screams and slams a door. You holler back at her. You don't understand what's happening or why she's so upset. Anger burns all the way down to her toes. She sobs. You roll your eyes because she's crying again and you're tired of it. She wants to knock those rolling eyeballs right out of your head. She needs to be understood and she doesn't think you're trying. You don't even know how to begin to try anymore. There is nothing you can do that is "right" in her eyes. There is nothing she can do to make it better. It's a pretty grim picture.

Men-take-pause.

You may feel like you're living with a distorted version of the seven dwarves: Itchy, Bitchy, Sweaty, Sleepy, Bloated, Forgetful and

Men – TAKE-O – Pause

Psycho. And, in essence, you are. Keep in mind that your job is not to change her or fix her, but merely to learn how to refrain from provoking her while you protect your marriage and love her through this.

You want her to be rational, but she can't. You want her to be happy, but she doesn't always know how. You no longer feel like you know how to make her happy. You want the woman you married back, but she doesn't exist anymore. You wonder how long you can live with this *Medusa* model of your wife, fearful that at any moment she'll turn you to stone. And if she could...well, let's just say there'd be a lot more lawn ornaments in suburbia USA.

Men -Take-O - Pause

So, how do you survive menopause when the very nature of it can be irrational and erratic?

There is a logical strategy to soothe the menopausal beast, but it's not fail-proof and it will require a great deal of focus and commitment on your part. A solution exists but you have to go back to the very beginning of your relationship to find it.

In the beginning, you wooed her into falling in love with you. You were most likely more tolerant, more patient, more romantic, more positive, more tender and affectionate, more attentive and pursuant of her at any and all costs. In the beginning you were getting to know her and going the extra mile to ensure that her emotional needs were being met. To her, your attention was a barometer of your feelings. That attention was how you won her heart in the first place, and that's how you can win the real her back now.

It is the natural course of any relationship that over time romance dwindles. Love grows deeper and stronger, but outward affection and attention often falls by the wayside. Life gets in the way. Work. Kids. Family. Obligations. Sadly, by the time we meet the demands of everyone else around us, we often have little energy left for our spouse.

When menopause hits, that lack of affection and lack of attention that has otherwise not seemed to bother her, becomes magnified.

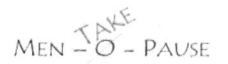

She suddenly feels unwanted, unloved, unnoticed, unappreciated and alone. You may not have altered your behavior at all, but menopause has altered her perception of it.

This isn't your fault. Nor is it hers. Her perception, now tweaked by menopause, is her new reality. It's not *your r*eality, it's hers and unfortunately you cannot change that no matter what you say or do. The best you can do is play by the new rules of her menopausal mindset and re-learn how to show your love.

You can do this by going back to the beginning and re-pursuing her. You have to think in terms of proving yourself all over again because right now she's seeking change.

MEN -TAKE- O - PAUSE

Don't let the thing she changes in her life be you because you clung to your rigid reality instead of meeting her in the midst of hers.

We all know men and women are different. To over simplify those differences, we could say that men are easier to satisfy because their needs can be met in physical ways. For example, you've heard the adage, "the way to a man's heart is through his stomach." Many men feel loved when a woman cooks for him. Most men feel loved through sexual intimacy and time spent together.

Problems often arise because men and women tend to define quality time differently. Men think quality time is time spent together,

MEN -TAKE- O - PAUSE

thus, they are fulfilled. Women think quality time is the time in which his focus is one hundred percent on her. Thus, she is often unfulfilled. This can be confusing for a man because in your reality you have spent hours together; but in her reality you have not been together at all.

Let me give you an example to help you understand. Being in the same room while watching a football game is not quality time to a woman. It's time together, which fulfills your need, but there is no quality to it, so she is left lacking. Watching you scream at the TV doesn't warm her heart or make her feel loved. It may be a fun activity, but it does not fill her need for quality time.

MEN - TAKE - O - PAUSE

You might be shaking your head right now and throwing up your hands, thinking you'll never understand how to please her. *What does she want already?!*

Women need to feel desired and sought after. She needs to see you actively choose her above all else, the way you did when you first met. She needs your undivided attention, not have you glancing at your phone or at the television while she's talking. She needs you to hold her hand for no reason at all. Most of all, she needs to know that she matters.

She needs to know that what is important to her, matters to you.

MEN -TAKE-O - PAUSE

She needs to know that you will listen and hear her. She needs to see you defend her, support her and always have her back, even when you disagree with her perspective. She wants to know that you will put in the effort for her, not just choose the easiest route. She needs to know you will not abandon her.

You might be thinking, *Oh, is that ALL?!*

No, there's more. In menopause, now more than ever, she needs you to fight for her and for your relationship because right now she is incapable of fighting for the marriage. Everything in her body is working against her. She feels trapped. Stuck. Backed into a corner by the circumstances of her own existence. Everything in her is screaming for freedom and change.

Men – Take – O – Pause

How do you fight for her when it feels like all she is doing is fighting against you?

The first and most logical way is to speak to her in *her* love language, *not in yours.* The statistical probability that you have spent years speaking to her in *your* love language instead of hers is very high. In fact, it's the number one relational error humans make. We all too often opt for the easiest way instead of the best way. I like to use the bag of chips analogy to explain this. Let's say you're having guests over for a bar-b-que. The easiest thing to do is open the bag of chips and set it on the table. The best thing to do is take the time to empty the bag of chips into a bowl and place the bowl on the table. It looks nicer and shows your guests that you invested a little thought and time into preparing for them.

Most of you are contorting your faces into confused expressions right now. You're thinking, *what's wrong with putting a bag of chips on the table?* Nothing's wrong with it. It's fine. But, let me ask you this: Do you want your marriage to be *fine* or do you want to make it *great*? Because sometimes the difference between *fine* and *great* lies simply in a little extra effort.

It's like opening a bottle of wine and being faced with two choices. You can either pour the wine into wine glasses or you can chug directly from the bottle. Both scenarios provide wine, but pouring it into wine glasses shows the extra effort that makes all the difference.

What the menopausal woman needs is to see you going the extra mile and making the extra effort to speak to her in her love language. She needs you to put the proverbial chips in a bowl instead of just throwing the opened bag on the table. She needs to sip wine from a glass and not have to swig from the bottle.

You may think you've done a fabulous job at showing her love through the years. But it is probably closer to the truth to say that you've done a fabulous job at *trying* to show her love. Up until now she's been able to give you credit for those attempts, even when they were not in her heart's language. She was able

Men TAKE-O-Pause

to give you points for trying and for all of the niceties that came with it. But that credit was temporary and accrued little interest because it was not in *her* heart's currency; but, rather, in yours.

The menopausal woman is no longer able to give you credit for those gestures. She now sees them as selfish. She sees them as a direct and conscious denial of her needs. Worse yet, she begins to believe that you think she isn't worth the extra effort.

This causes great dissention in marriages. The man becomes angry and accuses the woman of being unappreciative of all that he does for her. The woman grows defensive and upset because she isn't unappreciative, she's just tired of feeling unfulfilled and having her heart's needs blatantly ignored.

Men-take-pause. Remember, her perception is the new reality in which you both dwell. It may not be rational, but it is nonetheless real.

Let me give you a physical example: Let's say that she needs a fork. Perhaps she has even verbalized the need for a fork. Instead of giving her a fork, you come home and you give her one hundred spoons. You display the spoons beautifully and they are shiny and clean. You say, "Look at what I have given you because I love you." She thanks you for the spoons and quietly retreats to hide her brokenness. You see, you didn't care about her need. You didn't hear her heart. You

MEN -TAKE-O - PAUSE

didn't fulfill her. You loved her in the manner in which *you* saw fit. You didn't love her in the way *she needed* to be loved. Therefore, her heart was left empty. She needed one fork and a hundred spoons could not fill the void only the fork could fill.

Every time you choose to love her in your way instead of her way, she is instantly placed in a lose-lose situation. If she complains about the spoons, you call her unappreciative and ungrateful. So, she must pretend to love the spoons and suppress her need for the fork. She's been able to pull off this pretense until now.

The menopausal mindset no longer allows for the suppression of needs. Menopause demands those needs are met.

Give her the fork or you just may wind up with a hundred spoons shoved up your ass. That's her new outlook.

How do you love her the way she needs to be loved? How do you give her the proverbial fork?

Everyone has a unique love language which is usually a combination of five elements: words of affirmation, quality time, acts of service, receiving gifts, physical touch. If you don't know what her love language is then you are incapable of speaking to her heart; and if you're not speaking to her heart then you are wasting your time and energy because you're no longer getting credit for your actions. It really is that simple.

MEN -TAKE- O - PAUSE

Deciding to speak someone's love language or deciding not to speak someone's love language is an active, conscious choice and the menopausal woman is holding you accountable for that choice. She's calling you to the carpet. It's go-time. All cards on the table. If you don't speak her language, you will not get points or credit for the niceties done in your own language. That's the new deal. That's the menopausal mindset.

Fighting against that mindset will only result in the deterioration of the marriage. The reason is, she can't control it. She's not purposefully trying to make your life more difficult. She's simply trying to feel better and the only way she can imagine feeling better is in feeling loved, valued, appreciated and known. You bear this burden because no one else can fulfill her deepest needs, but you.

Menopause is your chance to be the hero she deep-down believes you are.

This shouldn't be a battle of wills. She needs you now more than ever, and if that means you have to push away your ego, or acquiesce to what you deem is illogical thinking, isn't she worth the effort? Let me help you with this one, the answer is YES!

When you choose to love her your way instead of her way, what that tells her, loud and clear, is that she is *unworthy* of your time, effort and affection. It breaks her heart every single time it happens. That's not something you can take back or kiss and make all better. That's something that scars the heart forever.

Don't let scar tissue destroy your marriage. Men-take-pause.

Don't waste your time loving her in your ways, where you get no credit. Start loving her in *her* way, where you get full credit and accrue life-long interest. This is the logical solution. This is what makes you the hero of her heart. This is how you quiet the menopausal monster and keep your wife grounded in the stability of your affection. This is how you survive menopause together.

Let me give you some simple examples. If her love language is words of affirmation but you are coming home with flowers and candy and taking her to fancy restaurants, you're not speaking to her heart. You may be making romantic gestures and doing nice things, but you're not loving her *in the way she needs to be loved.* You're loving her in the way that fits your definition of affection; not hers. This equates to a selfish love, not a selfless one and the menopausal woman sees right through it.

If her love language is quality time and you send her beautifully written cards but never give her your undivided attention, you are not speaking to her heart. Instead, you are pushing her further away. When she comes to you and complains that you never spend time with her and you say, "But I give you beautiful cards," your words are meaningless. It's the equivalent of taking your car into the shop to get the oil changed and instead they fill it with gas. You complain, stating, "I needed an oil change." To which they shrug and say, "You should be more appreciative because I filled your tank with gas." The gas is fine, but you still didn't get what you needed.

If you lavish her with acts of service, from setting the table to scrubbing toilets and doing the laundry, but her love language is receiving gifts, you have fallen short of loving her heart. She'd rather have dirty toilets than feel unworthy of being loved.

Real love is not defined as taking the most convenient or easiest road. It is often taking the rocky path less traveled. It is doing whatever is necessary, at whatever cost, even if it is uncomfortable, to show your affection.

MEN - TAKE - O - PAUSE

Remember, to her, your effort is a barometer of your affection. If you don't take the time to speak to her in *her* love language, you will ultimately make her feel unworthy of being loved.

Deciding to love her, *her* way will not go unnoticed. The points you accrue in this account generate interest forever.

The pre-menopausal woman, with the buffer, could issue credit for kind gestures even if they weren't in her love language because she was younger, had more room to store suppressed needs and a more viable outlook to maintain peace and hold the relationship together.

The menopausal woman with no buffer no longer has the ability to offer partial credit;

MEN ~~TO~~ JAKE - PAUSE

nor does she want to. She believes she deserves more. She deserves to be loved in the manner in which she needs to be loved, not in the way that is easiest or most comfortable for you. She no longer cares about peace or what's fair and she no longer has room to suppress unmet needs.

Her hormones have raised the bar. She doesn't want your spoons. She wants a fork! Screw the gas you put in the car, she needs a friggin' oil change! You can no longer get away with doing things your way. You can no longer make substitutions and get credit. Now, you have to do it according to *her* definition of what is "right."

And "right" is defined as meeting the standards of her heart, not the standards of your rational convenience.

The way in which she needs to be loved and feel loved may not be rational in the context of your logic. But keep in mind that this really isn't about you; it's about her. You have to decide what's more important to you, your finite thinking or the condition of her heart? Your rigid reality or the fulfillment of her soul? Remember, you're living in the reality of her perception now, not yours.

Every time you attempt to love her your way instead of *her* way, you show her that you don't *really* care. You show her that at the end of the day, as long as you have done what you deem to be your husband-type duties of providing for the family, you don't really give a damn whether she feels loved or not. This causes irreparable damage to the relationship.

That may not be how you feel at all. In fact, that may be the furthest thought from your mind. But, that is her perception of your actions.

It's not rational. It's not logical. It's never going to make sense to you. But that doesn't make it any less real to her.

The menopausal beast is watching and with every action you are either proving that your way of thinking and your way of doing things is more important to you than her, or you're showing her that you'll sacrifice any and every rigid notion you have to make her feel adored. There is no in-between. There is no gray area. She is either loved or not. You either care or you don't. The menopausal mindset is black and white.

If you want to calm the nagging, menopausal beast then you must speak to that beast in the language in which it can understand. You have the power to soothe the menopausal monster but you have to make the choice to put in the time and effort, realizing that there is no room for short-cuts anymore.

Men-take-pause. You must show her that you are in this battle together and that you are strong enough to hold the reins while the menopausal beast bucks and kicks.

MEN – TAKE/O – PAUSE

#9

"Menopause… a pause while she reconsiders men."

CHAPTER NINE

She'll Get Over It, Right?

"She'll get over it, right?" Men ask about menopause with trembling hearts and fear-stricken eyes. Eventually, yes, but just as hurricane winds eventually subside, the real question isn't when will the storm end but how much damage will it leave behind?

In a recent survey conducted by AARP magazine, "over 60 percent of divorces are initiated by women in their 40s, 50s or 60s." This is because something in their brain disconnects and they no longer have the drive to communicate and work things out. They're suddenly more prone to walk away than they were years prior. They're no longer willing to settle and sacrifice if they don't feel like their needs are being met, emotions validated and commitment to the relationship reciprocated. If they're already feeling alone in the marriage then they have less fear of being alone outside of it.

Men-take-pause.

It is imperative that you understand what is happening in her brain and realize that she can't just "get over it."

Don't stick you head in the sand and simply plan to wait out the storm. By the time you emerge, she will be gone. Your inability to withstand the storm and prove your love will

MEN –TAKE–O – PAUSE

have damaged the marriage beyond repair. You'll blame her because she changed but the fault will be yours because you refused to change with her. See, her change isn't a choice. It's happening *to* her. Your change or refusal to change is an active choice. Don't make this mistake.

You're not just battling a bitchy woman with mood swings. You're fighting a chemical beast with sharp teeth and claws.

You know that "for better or for worse" contract you signed on your wedding day, well, this is where the rubber meets the road.

When a woman's estrogen level drops something in her brain snaps, suddenly recalling to conscious memory every grudge she's ever held. Every time you offered spoons instead of the fork she needed, now consumes her with anger and injustice. She becomes destabilized, as she feels that everything in her life is coming unglued, making her prone to irrational, life-altering decisions. She wants change and even if she can't define exactly what that means, she's willing to do just about anything to embrace it.

What's more is the fact that she no longer possesses the ability to suppress dissatisfaction going forward. In other words, she's going to call you out on your shit. In fact, she's going to call everyone in her life out on their shit. She now lives by the motto, "the squeaky wheel gets the oil." This means that she's going to squeak and squeak and squeak.

If you make a conscious decision not to provide oil, take cover because a storm is coming.

Medically speaking, when estrogen levels drop, levels of oxytocin, which is a feel-good hormone attributed to feelings such as love for others, and the urge to take care of one's family, also drop. This is why menopausal women often suffer from bouts of sadness and even depression.

Some doctors claim that the lack of oxytocin changes a woman's thinking from a WE mindset to a ME mindset, hence making it easier for her to erratically end a long-term friendship or relationship.

Adding to the hormonal aspect is the fact that many menopausal women have spent much of their lives caring for other's needs and

MEN -TAKE-O - PAUSE

sacrificing their own desires in the process. Many have given up careers to raise children or to care for elderly parents. Many have moved away from family and friends in support of their spouse's career. Many are now in the midst of empty-nest syndrome and are already trying to re-define what their lives look like. Don't let her re-write the story of her life without you in it.

Menopause not only magnifies her sacrifices but intensifies her desire to have her own needs met.

If you don't meet her needs, she'll subconsciously search for something that will because at this point, unfulfillment is no longer an option.

Much like how the biological fertility clock of a woman in her thirties ticks to procreate, the menopausal woman is keenly aware that time is running out. She will often ponder, *when is it my turn to be happy?*

The correct answer is now. NOW is her turn to be happy. And the correct catalyst for finding that path to happiness is you. This is your job as her husband and it's a good job because if you do it right, you'll be her hero.

What you need to hang onto through this process is the fact that menopause is temporary. In time, her body will rebalance. Your job is to ensure that her chemical imbalance doesn't blow up your marriage in the short-term. You can't do that if you hide or run away. You can't do that if you cling to your ego. You can't do that if you choose to love her *your* way instead of *her* way. If you give up now, the relationship will not survive. The menopausal her doesn't have the tools to save the marriage.

Sadly, too many women end up having affairs and/or spontaneously filing for divorce during the menopausal years. In a recent poll, the top two reasons women in their 40s, 50s and 60s stated as reasons they left their husbands were (a) he took me for granted (meaning she felt unloved and unappreciated), and (b) he refused to change.

As her husband, you have the power to protect your marriage from such a tragic end.

MEN -O - PAUSE *(JAKE written above O)*

Knowing that menopause will not last forever, you can make the conscious choice to temporarily change with her, to alter your perspective to fit her present needs no matter how illogical it may seem, and ultimately save your relationship.

The number one reason men filed for divorce in their 40s, 50s and 60s was lack of sex, which is not surprising since a low-libido is a common symptom of menopause.

It begs the question, if those men had realized that her low-libido was chemical and not necessarily indicative of her heart for him, would they have been more patient? Was the marriage worth enduring a temporary lack of sexual drive, knowing it would get better in the long-run? My guess is, yes.

Men-Take-O-Pause

A low-libido can be frustrating for both the man and woman. It's okay for a man to feel agitated by this because it isn't fair to him. But it's not okay for a man to spew snide comments and make resentful remarks that pressure her with guilt and make her feel that much more of a failure.

Keep in mind, menopause is something that happens *to* her. But how you handle it is an active choice and you bear the long-term burden of that choice.

The change in her is chemical and beyond her control. If she could snap her fingers and feel turned on and ready for action, she'd do it. If she could make your touch feel pleasing again, she would. She misses the intimacy. She misses the craving. She misses

Men – TAKE – O – PAUSE

you and she hates that sex has become a wall between you. But she is powerless against her own body and she needs to know that the condition of her soul is more important to you than sex.

What it boils down to is that you get to decide what comes first. Her heart or your dick?

Menopause isn't fair; not to you and not to her. It's a monster that wants to chew up your marriage and spit it out. But you hold the key to controlling the monster. Every time you make the active choice to love her the way she needs to be loved, you are soothing the beast. Every time you consciously decide to embrace her emotional perspective instead of rigidly gripping your own logic, you are creating calm.

Each time you validate her instead of trying to fix her or change her, you are proving that you have the strength to withstand the storm. You're proving that you're her hero and that she is not alone.

In the darkest moments, when you become frustrated and think you cannot stand another mood swing or complaint, or when the temptation to find sexual satisfaction elsewhere enters your mind and you justify it by her frigidity…

Men-take-pause.

Step back. Look at the past and recall all of the times she has put out for you and put up with you. Now, it's your turn.

Paybacks are literally a bitch.

MEN -TAKE-O - PAUSE

#10

"Let's talk about sex, baby. Let's talk about you and me."

CHAPTER TEN

Conquering the Low Libido

We've already talked about avoiding the menopausal booby traps, now let's talk about how to get more booby time.

A low libido can have drastic effects on any relationship. It can be devastating. But it is also something that can be overcome if you and your spouse work together. A low libido doesn't have to be a reason to stop engaging in sexual intimacy. In the words of Rick Springfield, "We all need the human touch."

This need is powerful and should not be overlooked.

Women who suffer from low libido don't just manifest physical symptoms. Far worse than the physical ramifications is the underlying emotional toll. The menopausal woman with a low libido subconsciously attaches a sense of guilt to sex. She knows her husband wants sex and she feels guilty by the fact that she suddenly has no desire to fulfill him. This lack of desire then garners fear that eventually he will seek fulfillment elsewhere.

Thus, sex that used to represent love, fun, spontaneity and intimacy now represents guilt, fear and often times physical pain. I don't have to tell you that this is a pretty bleak picture.

So, how do you remain intimate during menopause, when everything in the woman's body is working against it?

Once again, it's time to tweak the perspective and be open to change.

It is not uncommon for couples who have been together for a long time to settle into a same 'ol, same 'ol approach to sex. During menopause, *the Get-On, Get-In, Get-Off, Get-Out, Get-Off* routine may no longer work. Menopause is the time to think outside the box.

Sexual intimacy is not just about intercourse. In other words, the only thing *missionary* about your approach to sex should be that you're on a *mission* for intimacy.

There are many, many ways to be intimate. The most important component of sexual intimacy is touch. People need to feel the warmth of another person. Their breath on your neck, their fingertips against your skin, the tenderness of their lips enclosing on yours. We all have an innate need for closeness and this need cannot be ignored without causing damage to the relationship.

Communication is paramount. It's important to address the issue of sex from a "we" perspective instead of a "me" perspective. What I mean by this is that you don't want to sit down and tell her why *you* need sex. She knows why you need it. In addition, you don't want to remind her of how long it's been since you've had sex. Again, she

Men – TAKE – O – Pause

already knows. Hearing you talk about your sexual needs will only intensify her guilt and prompt a defensive response.

You will want to address it from a "we" tone, emphasizing that you are in this boat together and finding a way to bridge the intimacy gap will strengthen your marriage.

First and foremost, have a detailed discussion about the physical components of sexual intimacy and find out what no longer feels good to her. Remember, the menopausal woman's body is ever-changing and what she liked yesterday may not be what feels good today. You're going to need to be flexible and roll with the changes if you want consistent booby time.

Men -Take-O - Pause

For example, during menopause some women experience vaginal dryness to the point that intercourse becomes extremely painful. If this is the case, talk about adding lubricants to your routine or place more emphasis on oral sex for a while. Some women experience severe breast tenderness, to the point that even the slightest touch to the nipple can be painful. If this is the case, discuss alternative forms of touching, including breast massage that doesn't involve fondling the nipple. Some women develop an overly sensitive sense of smell and taste that makes French kissing nauseating. If this is the case, discuss brushing teeth right before kissing so both mouths are clean and minty fresh.

Men - Take-O - Pause

Whatever the case may be, seeing that you are willing to accept the changes in her body and fine-tune your approach will help her realize that she is not alone in this. It will help her understand that this is not a you-against-her-fight, but rather, it's the two of you battling the chemical beast together. Knowing that you are not blaming her or resenting her for having a low libido, will relieve her sense of guilt, help her relax and make her more emotionally available for intimacy.

Second, discuss making a commitment to one another to bomb the beast by engaging in intimacy several times per week. Again, emphasize that it's not just for *you*, but for her and for your marriage as a whole. The menopausal monster wants to make her feel

MEN – TAKE – O – PAUSE

isolated, alone and unloved. Intimacy is the key to destroying the monster. A weekly dose of intimacy minimizes the menopausal woman's guilt over not fulfilling her husband's needs, reduces her feeling of failure and curtails the fear that he will seek gratification elsewhere. It literally lightens her load and frees her mind. It's a win-win-win. A win for him. A win for her and a win for the marriage.

Third, menopause has a way of stifling playfulness so discuss ways in which you can liven up your sex life.

This is middle-age, not the middle ages; explore new methods together.

Men Take-O-Pause

Buy sex toys. Some men are averse to dildos and vibrators, feeling as if they alone should be able to satisfy the woman in their life. But this self-inflicted pressure may no longer be realistic with all of the changes in her body. The truth is some women have great difficulty achieving orgasm during menopause. This can cause frustration for the man because a technique that was once fool-proof now falls short, making him feel inadequate. It can also become a huge source of physical and emotional frustration for the woman. So, for the sake of marital intimacy, you may need to lay aside any personal hang-ups you have with sex toys. There is no shame in using a vibrator with your wife. It doesn't mean your instrument of manhood isn't efficient or adequate. It simply means her body has changed and you are man enough to accept the change and tweak your technique. A side benefit of using a vibrator is that it's a lot less work for you and you still get credit for the end result. (wink)

Make-love in new places. Try new positions. Massage each other's hands and feet, shoulders and assess. Let your fingers reach in and touch your spouse's soul.

This sounds easy on paper, but make no mistake, it doesn't come without pitfalls. Here are some important things to be aware of:

Timing is everything.

Men, you must be intuitive enough to realize the difference between a good time to pursue intimacy and a bad time. There are right and wrong moments and you will need to pay close attention to her mood in order to ascertain the difference. During menopause it may seem like there are more wrong times than right. What you don't want to do is pursue sexual intimacy at the wrong moment, causing the menopausal mindset to spiral into guilt-laden depression or bringing on an all-out attack by the menopausal beast whose defenses you've awoken.

For example, when you see that she is having a rough day, that she is tearful or ranting, it is not the time to attempt sexual intimacy. When she tearfully buries her head in your shoulder in need of a hug, it is not the time to go in for a boob grab. In the middle of a hot flash is not the time to start massaging her breasts or grabbing her ass. In fact, during a hot flash the only attention she wants from you is for you to put a cold compress on the back of her neck and fetch her a glass of ice water. When she is thrashing around in bed, kicking off the covers and complaining that she is hot, that is not the time to climb on top of her and pursue sex. The only thing she wants from you at that moment is to open a window, turn on a fan or adjust the thermostat down several degrees.

So, when *is* the right moment? Watch for clues. For example, if you're sitting on the couch watching television, take her hand in yours and gently massage it. If she starts to massage your hand back, this is a good sign.

Move slowly and judge whether it's a good time or a bad time by the way she responds to your advances.

Don't take it personally when you're shot down.

The human ego is fragile and can be wounded when sexual advances are not reciprocated. Being shot down can make a person feel insecure and even angry. These are normal emotions and you shouldn't feel guilty for having them. After all, you're fighting to keep your marriage together and that fight during the menopausal years often feels one-sided and unfair.

When you feel this way, remind yourself that her lack of reciprocation isn't personal. Her body is working against her and against your advances. It doesn't mean you aren't still the man she deeply adores. It doesn't mean you are doing anything wrong. It simply means the beast has won this round; but you will win the war.

Make yourself appealing.

Keeping in mind the fact that the menopausal woman's senses are heightened and every flaw is highlighted, men are faced with a new challenge. In order to fulfil the most primal of urges, they must now find a way to attract their mate.

Men -Take-O- Pause

In long term relationships people settle into ruts and routines. Often times they stop dressing up for one another, stop shaving as often, and cease to do the little things that attracted each other in the first place. It is important to put those things back into your daily repertoire.

Let me give you some examples. For the menopausal woman who is already feeling ugly and fat and miserable, it is important for her mental and emotional health to put on her make-up, fix her hair, dress in an outfit she likes, get her nails done, shave her legs, wear perfume, etc. It is emotionally beneficial for her to take outward steps to make herself feel inwardly better. She used to do these things for you, but during menopause it is important that she does these things for herself, as well.

Notice when she does. Compliment her appearance, her scent, her beauty. She may outwardly deny your words, but inwardly they will be treasured. Also, notice when she doesn't do these things because this can be a sign of lingering sadness transitioning into depression.

By the same token, it is important, now more than ever, that you make yourself look good for her. Dress the way you know she likes you to dress. Wear the cologne that you know she likes. Shave if she likes a clean-shaven face. Grow a beard if she likes a furry face. Look good. Smell good. These simple things will be

MEN –TAKE–O – PAUSE

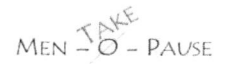

perceived as actions of affection and attention. You will score big points in her heart for them.

Go above and beyond and see what happens. Give her reasons to feel drawn to you. For example, put a dab of cologne in your private area just in case oral sex is on the docket. If she does begin a descent in the bedroom, she will notice and will feel loved by the action.

It's often the little things that mean the most and that make the other person feel noticed and appreciated.

Don't pursue sex, pursue intimacy.

Let intimacy lead into sex. If you chase after sex, her low-libido and the emotional attributes tied to it will crush you. If you patiently seek intimacy, you will slowly snuff out the menopausal monster's defenses and open her heart.

Let's face it, guys, when her heart opens her legs will follow.

MEN – TAKE / O – PAUSE

#11

"Menopause... if it doesn't kill you it will make you stronger."

CHAPTER ELEVEN

Talk is Cheap

The best thing you can do for the menopausal woman in your life and for your marriage as a whole, is cheap. In fact, it's absolutely free. Talk. Keeping the lines of communication open is crucial because there will be times for both of you when frustrations are high and tolerance is low. Being able to communicate in a non-confrontational, non-demanding way, even when she might be pointing a finger at you, will help ward off a full-blown argument.

Men – Take-O – Pause

Come to her with no solutions, just open arms.

This can be harder than it sounds because many men have the "Mr. Fix It" syndrome. You are biologically designed to want to fix things that are broken. Thus, menopause can be extremely frustrating for you. Many men feel as though they are failing when they can't make things better, but this is not the case with menopause. You are not failing.

Remember, she doesn't expect you to have the answers or be able to make everything better. She doesn't need you to fix it, she simply needs you to be strong enough to endure the storm with her.

Now that you know what she is experiencing chemically, emotionally and the associated thoughts that go with these changes, you can use this information to spark a conversation. The more you and she can discuss what is happening, the easier it will be for you to understand her mood swing triggers and navigate the menopausal landmines.

Remember, your job is to safeguard your marriage and you do that by protecting her heart.

Earlier in the book we talked about phrases that should never be uttered in the presence of a menopausal woman. Now, let's look at some of things she longs to hear from the man in her life.

- ➢ Let her know that you are aware that you cannot relate to what she is experiencing. Tell her that you're not going to try to pretend that you get it nor are you going to make light of it. Though you don't know what it feels like or what is happening, you're here for her and you're not leaving or giving up.

- ➢ Tell her that you see the changes in her and that you are willing to alter anything in your marriage and in your life to accommodate those changes.

Tell her that changing doesn't scare you, but losing her does.

➢ Tell her that you will not allow her to withdraw when she is hurting or shut you out. You will seek her out because you believe that you can work through this together. She is not alone and you won't let her be lonely.

➢ Acknowledge that you might not be as good at speaking her love language as you thought and promise to try harder to love her the way she needs to be loved. You no longer want to give her a hundred spoons when she's asking for a fork.

- As difficult as it can be, try to lay down your defenses because she will see strength in your humility. She will respect you more for being humble and open than if you try to pretend like there is nothing wrong.

- Tell her that it makes you sad to see her hurting and that it is frustrating when you can't fix this for her.

- Reassure her that if there is a temporary lull in your sex life, due to her low-libido, that you will work through it together and not seek sexual fulfillment elsewhere. You will pave a new road and keep intimacy between you.

MEN -TAKE-O - PAUSE

- ➢ Remind her that menopause is temporary and that eventually the darkness will lift.

- ➢ Ask her to stay open with you and to let you know when she is battling depression or feelings of sadness.

- ➢ Remind her that marriages survive menopause every day and that you intend to ensure that yours will survive as well.

- ➢ Tell her that you are committed to finding new ways to have fun together and to see her laugh more times in the day than she cries.

These are just a few suggestions of things that will soothe her heart. There are undoubtedly more examples and I am certain you can come up with some excellent ideas on your own. Try not to get discouraged if and when well-intended gestures blow up in your face. Trying something is always better than giving up or doing nothing. The reality is, if anyone has a shot at soothing her heart, it's you.

Keep in mind that your overall job as her husband, especially during menopause when her chemistry is fighting against you, is to fight for the woman you love and protect your marriage. Your job is not to fix her, because you can't; but to validate who she is and what she is going through. Love her in the way she needs to be loved. Be her light in the darkness when she fumbles around trying to find herself. Be the stability she lacks.

Marriage is a give and take union but in menopause, men must take pause and learn to give in ways that may be uncomfortable and in which you may be unaccustomed. You have to learn to speak the foreign language of her heart. It isn't easy.

Life isn't fair and menopause is even more unfair. It's cruel. It's agonizing. It's ugly. And it can be terrifying for both of you.

For men, it may feel like you're losing the woman you love. You may feel lonely, frustrated, angry and confused. You may want to reach for her but it feels as if every time you try, you're doing something wrong. Men-take-pause. Stop banging your head against a wall by doing the same things over and over. Instead, discover what her definition of "right" is and reach for her in that manner; even if it is illogical.

For her, it feels like the whole world is falling apart. Her self-esteem has flatlined. Her self-confidence is non-existent. She's a stranger in her body, in her home, in her marriage. She feels dormant, unknown even to herself, unnoticed by others, unappreciated by those close and unworthy of love in the way that she needs it.

As the ground cracks beneath her feet, grab onto her and hold tight. Carry her back to solid footing. Love her even when she's nagging at you. Be bigger and stronger than

MEN – TAKE – O – PAUSE

the beast. Be the hero of her heart because deep down, despite what she might utter in a menopausal rage, that's who she believes you are. That's why she married you in the first place. The beast only wins if one of you gives up. So, strap yourselves in, roll with the changes and ride this thing out together...

that's how you survive menopause.

~

Now, if you decide that this is all a bunch of bullshit and you feel no need to heed my advice, allow me to offer one final suggestion: Run. Hide. Sleep with one eye open. Because the menopausal beast will not rest until she eats you and your marriage alive.

Men-take-pause.

MEN – TAKE – O – PAUSE

ABOUT THE AUTHOR

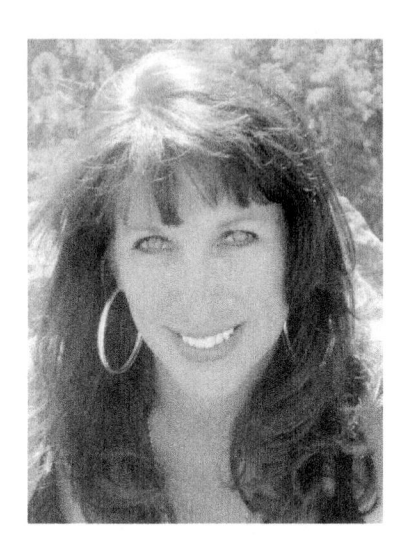

Susan Claridge, also writing under the penname S.R.Claridge, is a suspense writer, nominated for the 2010 Molly Award, 2013 Pushcart Prize and awarded the 2011 Rocky Mountain Fiction Writers Pen Award. She is most known for her thrilling mafia suspense series entitled, Just Call Me Angel. She loves autumn, moonlight and Grey Goose martinis with bleu cheese or jalapeno stuffed olives. She believes Friday nights are for indulging in Mexican food and margaritas and Sunday mornings warrant an extra-spicy Bloody Mary. Growing up in St. Louis, Missouri and earning her BA in Psychology from the University of Missouri, Columbia, S.R.Claridge is a mixture of mid-western family values and western wild nights. She loves Jesus, believes in the power of prayer, in the freedom of forgiveness and that life is a gift that should be enjoyed to the fullest. With a background in theatre, S.R.Claridge creates characters with dramatic flair and is known for her intense plot twists and engaging humor. S.R.Claridge would rather walk dangerously where there's a view than sit in idle safety and let life pass her by. Her spirited outlook comes shining through in her novels, as she takes readers to the edge of their seats with bone-chilling suspense.

You can learn more about the author and her books at www.SusanClaridge.com

Men -TAKE-O- Pause

BOOKS BY S.R.CLARIDGE

JUST CALL ME ANGEL series:

Tetterbaum's Truth *(book 1 in the Just Call Me Angel series)*

Traitors Among Us *(book 2 in the Just Call Me Angel series)*

Russian Uprising *(book 3 in the Just Call Me Angel series)*

Death Trap *(book 4 in the Just Call Me Angel series)*

Loose Ends (*book 5 in the Just Call Me Angel series*)

Divine Intervention *(book 6 in the Just Call Me Angel series)*

False Truths *(book 7 in the Just Call Me Angel series)*

Petals of Blood *(short story; Pushcart Prize Nomination 2013)*

House of Lies (*Political cult suspense*)

No Easy Way *(debut novel; nominated for The Molly Award from the HODRW 2010)*

The Candy Shop *(Suspense Thriller)*

** S.R.Claridge has also ghostwritten ten novels.

MEN -JAKE- PAUSE

AUTHOR ACCLAIM

"The Just Call Me Angel series is suspense at its best."

- RipeReviews

"A unique series from a one-of-a-kind author."

- APEX Reviews

"Riveting!"

- TrueBlueEbookReview

"One thrilling moment after another!"

- CanadaReviews

"A best-seller candidate indeed."

- BookWatchMagazine